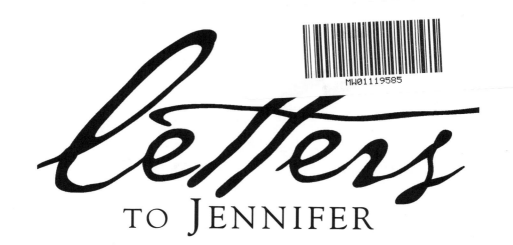

Letters

TO JENNIFER

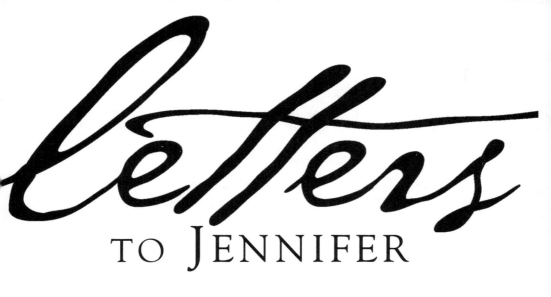

letters
TO JENNIFER

Sharon Gray

Oliver & Maudie Gray

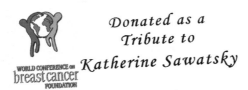

*Donated as a
Tribute to
Katherine Sawatsky*

WORLD CONFERENCE ON
breast cancer
FOUNDATION

Cover design and layout by Gallant Design Ltd.
Cover image by Tanja Berlin / Berlin Embroidery Designs (Tanja@berlinembroidery.com)

- Needlework of the cats was done with one thread of DMC cotton floss. Fourteen colours were used. The ground fabric is bone white Thai silk painted with silk fabric paints.

Book illustrations by Andrea Toews
Photographs provided by Sharon Gray
Printed and bound in Canada by Hignell Book Printing, 488 Burnell Street, Winnipeg, Manitoba Canada R3G 2B4 Toll Free: 800-304-5553

National Library of Canada Cataloguing in Publication

Gray, Sharon, 1942 -
Letters to Jennifer

Second Printing May 2008

ISBN 0-9686942-2-5

1. Gray, Sharon, 1942—Correspondence. 2. Johnston, Jennifer, d, 2002—Correspondence. 3. Breast—Cancer—Patients—Canada—Correspondence.

I.   Title.

RC280.B8 G72 2002   362.1'9699449'0092
C2002-9106303

Introduction

Jennifer and I met in the early eighties.

The first time she came to my home she met Basil and Sage, my two Siamese cats, and announced: "I am a dog person."

Over time she accepted them, particularly Basil. They frequently shared taco-flavoured tortilla chips on the kitchen floor.

She moved away, met Ted and married him. Ted was living with two gentlemen cats, Norman and Charlie. Of course, she became a "cat person."

We remained long distance friends. Over time we became employees of the same organization and Jennifer was my supervisor, living in another city. As Jennifer said, "Management by remote control." I was now living with Oliver and Maudie, two wonderful Siamese cats. At the time I was experiencing health difficulties and asked her if she would care for Oliver and Maudie if anything happened to me. She said that she would be delighted.

Whenever we met, she would ask: "And how are my niece and nephew?" Those who heard this would not realize that we were discussing two very precocious, charming cats.

In October 1999, Jennifer was diagnosed with breast cancer, had one breast removed and started on an odyssey of chemotherapy and radiation treatments. Christmas that year, a parcel arrived with Christmas presents, beautifully wrapped, for Oliver and

Maudie from "Auntie Jennifer." I was overwhelmed by this kind, thoughtful act. Of course, they had to write a letter of thank you to "Auntie Jennifer."

She told me she really enjoyed the Christmas thank you letter, therefore, the first of more than thirty Letters to Jennifer from Oliver and Maudie.

The letters were a non-threatening, non-evasive way of keeping in touch with her during this difficult time, and there was no need for her to reply. In humour, Oliver and Maudie describe their lives — living with Lip (live-in-person), their neighbours, events and generally their philosophy on life.

Jennifer — and others who have read them — urged that the letters be published and, for her they will be. Twenty percent of any profits will be given to Cancer Research and/or Cancer support organizations.

Cancer has touched all of our lives. Every day we hear of someone close or an acquaintance of someone we know who has been overwhelmed by this disease.

The poem by Natasha is about a relative of mine. Curtis died after a valiant battle with this disease. Christmas will always have a bittersweet resonance for us.

This book is for to everyone who has been affected by cancer.

ABOUT MAUDIE AND OLIVER...

November of 1993 I was living in a house without a cat.

After three weeks it was obvious to me this was not living. I started a search for two Siamese cats.

An advertisement in the local newspaper told of four Siamese kittens ready for homes. However, the phone number indicated that they were in the country. I called. The woman who answered the phone said that there were three males and one female. The female looked like the mother cat — lilac point — and her brothers were seal points, like the father cat. She also said that she handled them as much as she could so that they would be "people cats." This last statement made a trip to the country, in late November, necessary.

My best friend, Miriam and I started out on a Sunday morning in blizzard-like conditions. Miriam may not be a "cat person," but thankfully she is always ready for an adventure.

On the way, I told Miriam that I had already named the cats. The male would be "Oliver" and the female would be "Maudie."

We got hopelessly lost. After two phone calls from gas stations and some backtracking, we were on another snowy country road, inching our way along. A dark object on the side of the road became a farm dog, wagging his tail in greeting. He started down a driveway that was barely visible, stopped and turned. He was indicating to us that this is where we should be. He was right.

Inside, we were greeted by the mother cat, "Silver." Miriam gasped, "What a beautiful cat!" And she was.

The kittens were in a box in the kitchen.

The lady of the house handed me a small male kitten. He immediately leaned right into me and looked up with eyes and ears too large for his little face. He winked. A flirt, yet!

He then spoke: "Mrrriichk." I said he sounds like he has a speech impediment. "He will get over it," said the lady of the house. I thought: "I hope not." And he hasn't.

He then opened the door to my heart and, with his little paw, gave my heart a twist. It has remained twisted in Oliver's favour ever since.

It was apparent that Maudie, the female, was in charge as we watched her manage her brothers into subservience. She was perky and very full of herself. A potential beauty, with attitude. She showed the most tolerance for Oliver so I relieved her two other brothers of her tyranny. She is now as beautiful as her mother. Immediately, Maudie can sense a person in emotional pain and will show them great empathy and compassion. She is very loving and has a fondness for men as most of them allow her to flirt with them.

Just as we were leaving, with Oliver and Maudie in a cat carrier, I asked if we could see the father cat.

The lady of the house went to the top of the basement stairs and called, "Oliver!"

Acknowledgements

So many people had an influence on this endeavour — strangers that said something in a line-up at the market, acquaintances that said something that triggered a response, and friends with ideas.

I am grateful to you all. You are too numerous to detail here, but more important, I would regret it if I left someone out.

I thank you.

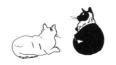

A Lost Battle

In Memory of Curtis A. Landega
January 1, 1981 — December 25, 2000

O, my beautiful older brother, as your life was sad,
It began on a day of enjoyment.
You tried your best; you went up a mountain,
You had fallen, but we didn't understand why.

Your doctor determined the severe problem,
You had cancer, are you going to die?
We all had fear, but we would also help you.
You were the most calm of us; did you want to flee?

You went everywhere for a cure,
A ray of light, a hope on the horizon.
Life will be more difficult for us.

But I know that you will be my beautiful saint.
I shall remember that you risked everything.
You lost; it is impossible that it is the end.

By Natasha Landega

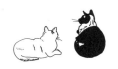

Une Bataille Perdue

En mémoire de Curtis A. Landega
Le 1ᵉʳ janvier 1981 — le 25 décembre 2000

O, mon beau grand frère, comme ta vie fut triste,
Il a commencé sur une journée de joie.
Tu essayas ton mieux, tu montas une piste,
Tu fus tombé, mais nous ne comprenions pourquoi.

Ton docteur détermina le sérieux problème,
Tu eus le cancer, est-ce que tu vas mourir?
Nous eûmes tous peur, mais on t'aiderait de même.
Tu fus le plus calme de nous, voulus-tu fuir?

Tu allas tout partout pour une guérison,
Un rayon de lumière, espoir à l'horizon.
La vie sera plus difficile pour nous.

Mais je sais que tu seras mon beau saint.
Je me souviendrai que tu risquais tout.
T'as perdu, c'est impossible que c'est la fin.

par Natasha Landega

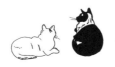

Table of Contents

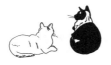

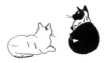

Letter #1 · Thank You for Christmas

December 28, 1999

Dear Auntie Jennifer:

We cannot tell you how pleased we
are with our Christmas gifts from you.

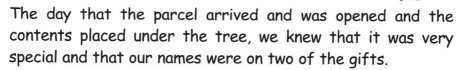

The day that the parcel arrived and was opened and the contents placed under the tree, we knew that it was very special and that our names were on two of the gifts.

This is Maudie speaking.

Lip is very strict about when the gifts are opened — can you believe — so we snuffed around and sorted our gifts from others so that there would be no delay on Christmas morning.

We opened the mice first and I have to tell you Auntie Jennifer, that Oliver is such an oaf about these mice. Immediately, he eats the tail off — and wonders why he is not "regular" for the next few days. This makes if very difficult for me to treat these horrid little mice things like they should be treated — grab the tail in my teeth, shake once then flip the mouse in the air over my shoulder. Now, this is no mean feat, as you can well imagine. It requires skill, endurance and timing. Of course, I am blessed with all of the above but Oliver's actions make it very difficult for me. So, I have become very adept at flinging the mice from the base of the tail. Same effect and I am pleased to tell you that they are now both a sorry sight, if I must say so myself. This is the way mice things should be treated.

Wow, were we surprised and pleased with the salmon cat candy! We never have candy so this has been absolutely delightful. Mind you, it is doled out on Lip's schedule, not ours. Needless to say, we have been very good over the holidays as it did not take us long to figure out the agenda for this item. She was very slow to open the box. We had to almost put it under her nose — she can sometimes be as daft as a brush. Of course, you know that because you work with her. We will continue to be paragons of virtue as long as the candy lasts — which will probably be quite a while.

Thank you so much Auntie Jennifer, we got the very best presents from you.

We wish you a very healthy and happy new year.

Lots of love,
Maudie and Oliver

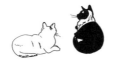

Letter #2 • Oliver is Goofy

January 7, 2000

Dear Auntie Jennifer:

Lip has just advised us that you are very ill and we are so sorry for this. Lip said that you were very sick last night and we hurt for you. We will pray for you to get all better. We pray a lot — meditate actually. This is of course when we are not grooming ourselves, which takes a lot of our time.

This is Maudie speaking.

I also help Oliver with his grooming, in particular his ears. Have you ever noticed how big his ears are? Don't know why, he never listens. He is having problems with his pee pee works again. He was whisked off to see Dr. Peter the other day — they didn't even tell me that they were leaving me ALL ALONE can you imagine. Sometimes they are so inconsiderate about me and my feelings.

Oliver has to take pills for his condition. YOW! Is he ever funny! He staggers around just after he has his pills and he has a glassy haze to his eyes — he is cross-eyed so it looks even more funny. (I'm not cross-eyed, I'm beautiful and lovely. But you know that.)

He does funny things too because of his pills. Two nights ago he hauled all his toys up onto the bed. This was no mean feat. He was quite exhausted after this. And, let me tell you, Lip was not amused! Imagine finding a wet dead mouse as a bedmate. We both had to scamper for safety! We thought that Lip would never return to normal.

Cleaning ladies came yesterday. This is quite a busy day for us as we must diligently supervise all of their actions. Imagine. Oliver, because of his goofy way, got more attention than I did. This is NOT a good thing.

We must sign off now, Auntie Jennifer, so that we can pray for you to get better.

Love,
Maudie and Oliver

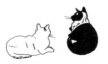

Letter #3 · We Do Hats

January 12, 2000

Dear Auntie Jennifer:

These two hats, and one that is still a WIP (work in progress) are from your friends in Cabin Safety. If you lose your hair, we do not want you to have a cold head and we feel you will look very chic in these. They were knit by Lip with great input and assistance from us.

This is Maudie speaking.

Since we were tiny babies we have been involved in the knitting process so we are now considered to be expert cat assistant knitters. Our job is whoever is sitting on Lip's lap, he or she must jump down and pick up any stitches that are dropped and return them to Lip. If green 100% wool stitches are dropped and Oliver is the assistant cat knitter, Lip sometimes does not get these back as he finds these very tasty.

The red hat knit is very large and it is big on Lip. We have threaded a piece of yarn through just under the rolled brim. Just untie it and adjust it as you want. We have included extra yarn for this.

The blue hat is of such a style that you will have to use pins if you get outside in a wind, or hang on tight!

Hope you enjoy these and the third hat will be forthcoming. It is not green so it will be a complete hat.

Love,
Maudie and Oliver

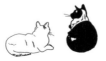

Letter #4 · Big Dust Up

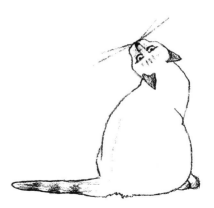

January 13, 2000

Dear Auntie Jennifer:

We had a big big dust-up last night.

This is Maudie speaking.

Lip and I went to bed very early last night as Lip had a new book. It was the twenty-second "The cat who..." book. The cat is actually two cats, Siamese of course, and their names are KoKo and Yum Yum. Koko and Yum Yum help their Lip solve all kinds of silly crimes that humans commit. Our Lip reads to us the parts about Koko and Yum Yum. They are some smart cats — sometimes smarter than the Lip they own!

I was in my usual spot when we first get into bed — just under the duvet cover in a comfortable position where I can see out and monitor what is going on. Oliver came to bed — finally — and brought one of the wet, sans tail mice. At this point Lip had fallen asleep — with the light on still holding the book. She does this often, you know. I was nodding off myself. Now Oliver starts to proceed under the duvet cover with wet slimy mouse. I hissed,

Lip awoke and told Oliver to take the mouse elsewhere. The light was turned out and all was quiet.

For a while.

Oliver came back with the mouse and started under the duvet cover with it clamped firmly in his mouth.

That is when I had to take control of the situation that was developing. I attacked him, wrestled him into a position where he cried "uncle." Lip awoke and there was a big dust-up. We were both sent scattering and had to find other sleeping accommodations for the night.

Of course, through all of this, where is the mouse? Well, it appeared this morning while Lip was fumbling around getting dressed. The mouse remained under the duvet cover and fell into the lower left corner of the cover which was on the floor. Lip stepped on it, screetched and carried on like you would not believe, Auntie Jennifer.

Well, we will never do that again, let me tell you! What a commotion! Auntie Jennifer, we were lucky that she remembered to feed us this morning.

Tonight there will be laundry. We are going to be very good and assist wherever we can, in particular making the bed. Most Lips do have a problem with this and it is important that we diligently assist in this area. We imagine that there will be an attempt to retrieve the mouse. We can help here too.

We will pray for you today Auntie Jennifer and we hope you are healing from the first chemotherapy treatment. Lip told us that this makes you very sick and very fatigued. We hope you will rest well and do nothing to make it any worse and do everything to make it better.

Love from
Maudie and Oliver(creep)

Letter #5 · Pigs Sing

January 18, 2000

Dear Auntie Jennifer:

This past weekend was very quiet, generally, for us as Lip was playing in a bridge tournament. When there is a bridge tournament, it is even quiet when Lip is here. She mumbles a lot about the behaviour and intelligence of her partners and it is not always nice so we will not repeat it here for you.

This is Oliver speaking.

As you know, Auntie Jennifer, I have been having problems again with my pee pee works. I have some new food that I find very appetizing — so does Maudie — and I take my pills twice a day. Lip tells me that I am the very best cat she knows for taking pills. I do not fuss, screech, run away — I open my mouth, the pill is put in and I swallow. When I am good about the taking of the pills I get lots of extra hugs and kisses. It is more important to have lots of hugs and kisses than to fuss about a pill, don't you think? I am feeling better now and I have only one pill left.

More stories about the duvet cover. As you know I hid Casper, the white mouse, in the duvet cover last week. The grey mouse is

Chester. Maudie and Lip don't even know their names. They treat the mice so shabbily and I get quite concerned for their safety. Maudie was getting set to cause bodily harm to Casper so I had to put him somewhere safe. It was only for a moment but then I forgot about him. Of course, Maudie had long forgotten about him as her attention span is somewhat limited to her fur, her nails, regular nap times, and of course, meals. Well, you know the rest of the story.

It is very difficult, Auntie Jennifer, to live with two assertive "skirts." My Uncle Sam moved away and took Auntie Betty with him. He doesn't visit me as often as he used to. He thinks that I need more male contact and he is probably right. Every time he comes over, we have man chats and I enjoy that very much.

I got sidetracked. I was telling you about the duvet cover. Last night everyone was very comfortable and sound, sound asleep. Lip and I woke to such a squeal like you have never heard before! Maudie fell down the side of the bed, inside the duvet cover. We were both standing on the floor before we realized that our darling Maudie was trapped and could not get out. What a todo!

Lip and I are now convinced that Maudie taught pigs to sing in one of her previous lives. Such a noise like you would not believe. Of course, she lost face and dignity over all this and it was not her fault, so she tells us.

Poor design, that duvet cover, with no respect for cats.

Last Friday before bridge I was assisting with the knitting while Lip and I watched the six o'clock news. One item was about a lot of flu going around in humans. It was recommended that everyone wash their hands thoroughly and often. I think it would be good for you to do that too, Auntie Jennifer, so that you do not get a cold or the flu. We cats do that often, so we think it is a good thing for humans, too.

I must sign off now for my nap number four.

All our love,
Oliver and Maudie

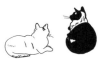

Letter #6 · Cleaning and Visits

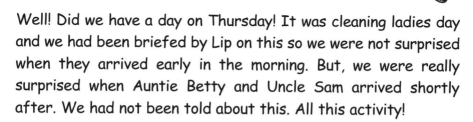

January 24, 2000

Dear Auntie Jennifer:

Well! Did we have a day on Thursday! It was cleaning ladies day and we had been briefed by Lip on this so we were not surprised when they arrived early in the morning. But, we were really surprised when Auntie Betty and Uncle Sam arrived shortly after. We had not been told about this. All this activity!

This is Maudie speaking.

Oliver was so hyper that he threw up on the living room rug. This was new to the cleaning ladies but not new to Auntie Betty.

She knew all about the special throw up cleaner and brush under the sink so she showed the cleaning ladies how to clean up spit-ups. I don't do this type of cleaning so I could do nothing.

You know, Auntie Jennifer, I just love men and I love Uncle Sam the most.

We went into the den and he let me sit with him on the chesterfield while he read.

While the cleaning ladies were making a lot of noise upstairs, Uncle Sam, Auntie Betty, Oliver and I sat in the living room with the fireplace on. It was a very lovely visit and we both received lots of love and petting. I don't think Uncle Sam and Auntie Betty get enough feline therapy since they moved away.

We love the cleaning ladies — Cindy and Cathy — and they are very kind to us. Cindy brushes me every time she comes. The brushings that I receive from Lip are very spotty, to say the least.

But, we think that the cleaning ladies actually make more mess than they clean up. First, they move all of our things around. This is most upsetting as our things are always where they are supposed to be. We try to get Lip to understand this but she too is less than satisfactory in this regard. Then the cleaning ladies start with the noise machine which usually sends us scattering.

This stirs up a lot of dust, at our level. Then, it settles back down again. It is very thick for a long time after they leave and we wander around in a low level dust storm for hours. This probably could be hazardous to our health.

It is time now for some grooming and then our major afternoon nap.

All our love to you, Auntie Jennifer and we are praying for you to get all better soon.

Love,
Oliver and Maudie

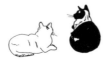

Letter #7 · Portraits of Us

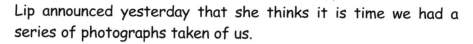

January 27, 2000

Dear Auntie Jennifer:

Lip announced yesterday that she thinks it is time we had a series of photographs taken of us.

This is Oliver speaking.

Immediately upon this announcement Maudie went into panic mode. (She is very vain and her beauty is very important to her.)

Maudie stated that she would have to have her nails done professionally.

Lip said that would not be possible as no Siamese Cat pedicurist within a hundred mile radius would do it as she has such a bad reputation and we are not driving out of town to some poor unsuspecting Siamese Cat pedicurist so that Maudie can put him/her into early retirement, probably with bodily harm and for certain, emotional trauma. Maudie will just have to do her nails by herself. I don't see what the problem is here as Maudie spends about two hours a day doing her nails, diligently.

Then Maudie wanted to know what colour for the background would we be using? It had better not be grey as she believes grey cannot possibly do justice to her abundant beauty. Lip said there is no grey in this house so relax, Maudie, we will not be using grey.

Lip asked what is your next concern, Maudie? I am sure we are not finished here. Maudie said that no, we are not. She said "You have been neglecting my grooming needs lately and I cannot remember the last time I was brushed." Lip replied " I brushed you last Saturday morning." "Phutz," said Maudie, "That was hardly a real brushing and I am going to have to be brushed for at least twenty minutes every day for one week before I could even consider having my picture taken. And, who will be doing the picture taking?" Lip replied that she would as a professional photographer may not survive the ordeal. Maudie said something unkind about Lip's photography skills that I will not repeat here, Auntie Jennifer.

This is Maudie speaking.

When Lip made an announcement about photo taking, Oliver became quite concerned about how he should pose for this. He has grey tummy hairs coming in and he is very self conscious about them.

I call them his grey pubic hairs and he blushes. Lip assured him that his grey hairs would not be photographed. Oliver wanted to know if he could be photographed with all of his toys — he is obsessed with the toys, Auntie Jennifer — his and mine. Lip said that would be taken into consideration. Oliver immediately started an intense grooming session and asked me to clean his ears. I said, "Oh after a while, I must nap now." I told him that it would take Lip some time to get her act together on this, so relax.

We will keep you informed about this, Auntie Jennifer and if there are any good pictures we will have Lip send them to you but don't hold your breath. We do love Lip but in some areas her skills are somewhat limited and this is one of them.

We were told you did not have your chemotherapy treatment yesterday because of your white blood cells. Please do healthy things to get them better and we are praying for you.

Love,
Maudie and Oliver.

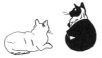

Letter #8 · Sleep In

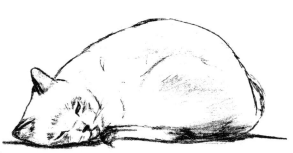

February 3, 2000

Dear Auntie Jennifer:

We have had two lovely days. Lip was home in bed and this is very special for us.

This is Oliver speaking.

When Lip is home in bed we are not shaken from the bed onto the cold floor before dawn but are allowed to cuddle up for long hours. A cat's delight! A human in bed producing warmth!

We take turns looking after her and never, never, do we leave her alone. Maudie is head nurse — she fits the profile perfectly. When she plays the role she sounds like a matron head nurse coming down the hallway and Lip and I say to each other "oh, oh, here she comes" and we sit up at attention.

Every so often Maudie bursts out in song. She does this when she is under the covers. That is when Lip calls her "Maudie MegaPurr."

I get to bring some of my toys to bed. They eventually get buried in the bed and turn up in places that seem to upset Lip. I think that Lip is not entirely happy with the new duvet cover but we think it is grand.

Lip has been working on a picture called "Retirement." Funny, we thought that retirement was a way of life — lifestyle — but what do we know, we are only cats, SIAMESE cats. We help her with this by sprawling on the chart. We put our left paw on the part of the chart she should be focusing on. After a while she says "Enough! I do know what I am doing!" Thank goodness she is a quick learner. We can then retire to the chesterfield for grooming or a numbered nap, whatever.

We have cleaning ladies today so there was no convincing Lip to allow us a sleep in. We must get our lists out and start our supervising duties. After we put our toys away.

Our toys are to be put away by four o'clock every afternoon and before the cleaning ladies come. As you can see, Auntie Jennifer, our lives are not that easy. I hate it when the toys are put away because I lose track of them and spend hours rounding them up again.

Lip told us that you had your second treatment yesterday. We hope and pray that it works well, and that the side effects are not too much for you to bear. We are always thinking of you.

Love,
Oliver and Maudie

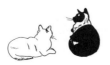

Letter #9 · Mice Bath

February 8, 2000

Dear Auntie Jennifer:

Well! Have we had another big dust-up in our lives. You will not believe!

This is Maudie speaking.

Sunday afternoon I was napping — afternoon nap #2 — after I had done my nails. Lip was out getting beaten to death at the bridge table.

Oliver had a plan and was diligently putting it all together. He collected all of the fur mice from around the house. There are a lot of fur mice around the house, Auntie Jennifer, — there are three white mice, two grey mice and a turquoise and yellow — quite ugly — mouse. Oliver then placed them all in the laundry basket. As you know, Oliver is the only attendant to the mice in this house — Lip and I have no use for them. We find them quite irritating and Lip is always mumbling when she comes across one and gently kicks it out of her path. I ignore them completely and put on my royal airs when I get near one.

Monday afternoon was laundry. Oliver and I participate in this process, particularly when the laundry first comes out of the dryer — we must inspect. We do this by climbing into the basket and burrowing down in the warmth. It is important to inspect it all. Very carefully. Lip does not understand this and we sometimes have to be strict with her so we can complete this important task to our satisfaction. Oliver and I share in this. We also share "assisting in making the bed" duties. If we persevere with this, we feel that Lip is eventually going to be a great bed maker.

Needless to say, all of the mice had a bath. That made them grossly unattractive — really ugly, Auntie Jennifer. Oliver is dumb, dumb, big time.

Well, when it was all over, it was very quiet. At least Lip dried them so they have returned somewhat to normal. Oliver got a big lecture. He took it very well — sat with his head bowed, through all the yelling. I hissed and told him "Oliver, you are dumb, dumb, big time."

I will be very kind- well, for a short time — to Oliver today as he is feeling very badly about all of this.

Maybe it a good thing that the mice had a bath, after all.

We hope you are feeling better. Eat well and get lots of rest, Auntie Jennifer.

Love,
Oliver and Maudie

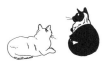

Letter #10 · Wise Like Danny

February 15, 2000

Dear Auntie Jennifer:

Lip has told us that she will be away for a week. We do not like this at all.

We are always well cared for by a whole lot of people but it is just not the same.

Because Lip was feeling guilty about this, she stayed home with us on Saturday night. That does not happen very often. We think that all of the theatres were closed and someone had stolen all the bridge cards for this to happen.

This is Maudie speaking.

We proceeded to the den and got Lip all set up with that stupid chart and "retirement" — the picture, not the lifestyle. Oliver and I settled on the chesterfield. Lip instructed us to listen carefully to Danny Finkleman on the radio as he is very wise and we may just learn something useful from him.

We even made a list for you, Auntie Jennifer, of all the things that he talked about so that you could become wise, also.

Here is the list:

"good fill at a party"

your show is irrelevant that is why you are still at CBC

low self-esteem (Danny, not us)

Cy, the Eaton's delivery man and his hat

valet parking at Eaton's

Policeman hats, baseball hats

no respect

increase in the number of channels, decrease in quality

you should mount binoculars on your lazyboy

periscope is needed to watch TV

slobbering on your chin

needed — better green garbage bags

zebras never let go

peas don't fly

brakes ABS

welcome is no problem

rocks fade to crystal

kids in political science stole the music

Italian food saves money

vacation at home like royalty

R & D hard candy

triple B kids don't play

too many adults

PROGRAM is hockey way.

Well, we are still working on this list and find it very difficult to become wise, to say the least.

We think that maybe Danny Finkleman is as daft as Lip. Maybe you can become wiser faster than we can, Auntie Jennifer.

We will not write to you next week as we will be busy telling and guiding our sitters on what, when and how we like to be cared for. Sitters create a lot of work for us.

Lip told us that you were planning on going skiing this week. We think this is wonderful. You be sure to dress warmly and wear your new hats. We know that you are scheduled for chemotherapy on the 23rd. We hope that your white blood cells are up to the right count and you will not be too sick after the treatment. We will pray for you, Auntie Jennifer.

Love,
Maudie and Oliver

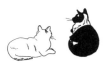

Letter #11 · We Are Lonely

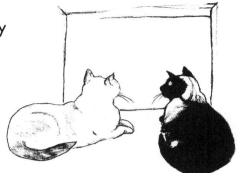

February 23, 2000

Dear Auntie Jennifer:

As you know, Lip was away last week. We do not like this at all. Uncle Sam and Auntie Betty dropped in twice to see us — they have such lovely tans as they just came back from Jamaica. Auntie Betty said that there were lots of cats where they were staying so they had lots of feline therapy while they were away.

This is Maudie speaking.

Auntie Sandra came every day but we can tell that she does not deal well with the basics of cat care. She has only had goldfish and they die. But, she does give us good loving and we are grateful for that.

We always try to get into Lip's suitcase when she is getting ready to leave us — heaven knows it is certainly big enough but she always tosses us out. We never know where she is going and we have no idea who is looking after her if we are not there. It is all very stressful this business of Lip leaving home.

After three days Oliver gets very anxious and decides to go and get Lip and bring her home. He starts by opening all the low drawers in the house. For reasons only known by Oliver, he feels he needs all of Lip's socks. They are all hand knit, Auntie Jennifer. He gets them all out onto the bedroom floor and then he goes to the TV cabinet and gets out the headset. He tells me he needs this to communicate with Lip. I asked him what the socks are for. He said he is still working on where they fit into all of this. After all this work a caregiver usually appears and puts all this stuff back and "talks" to Oliver. He bows his head and accepts his fate.

Now, if I were preparing for a trip like this I would do it quite differently.

First of all, I do not want to stray far from my luxurious creature comforts if I cannot take them with me. I would pack up all the food in the house, the green plaid chair (ideal for nap number 3), our basket in the closet with the custom made quilt, several towels, the hideabed from the den, the fireplace and of course, kitty litter facilities to last a lifetime. Oliver says I would impede his plan so that is why he does not ask me to accompany him. Ok by me. He is so weird.

Lip finally came home on Friday and we are now back to normal.

We were told you did not have your chemotherapy treatment on February the 23rd. We are so sorry about this as we are looking forward to the end of the chemotherapy as we understand that you might then come and see us. We would really like that, Auntie Jennifer. We are praying for you to get the white blood cells up to where they should be.

Love,
Oliver and Maudie

March 6, 2000

Dear Auntie Jennifer:

We have heard that you will be back to work this week. We are very pleased with this news.

This must mean that you are feeling better. Wonderful.

This is Oliver speaking.

Maudie has advised Lip and me that she believes that she is a "princess cat" and that she plans to live her life accordingly from here on.

Lip and I do not think that this is news but we are surprised that Maudie thinks it is news.

Maudie has acted like she is royalty from the day that she was born. I know, because I was there as I was born on the same day.

She has demanded that all the loose pillows on chesterfields be placed in the flat position and these will become her "princess cat thrones." She will take naps (number 3 and 4) on these pillows. I can join her but I must not share the throne as I am her lowly knave. I can nap below the pillow but I must not disturb the pillow, as that will disturb Maudie and we can't have that.

Maudie has demanded that Lip get her act together on the brushing. Maudie says that if she is to look like a "princess cat" she has to have additional and better grooming assistance from Lip. Lip is not so sure about this. She is going to phone Uncle Sam and see if he will be able to assist here. God knows that Maudie has already taken great advantage of Uncle Sam — since she was a baby! So this might go nowhere.

One day a long time ago, it was very hot and muggy. I was stretched at the open patio door attempting to direct a cool breeze over my very warm body. Uncle Sam came to the door and stepped in for a brief chat with Lip. Maudie, with her big crush on Uncle Sam and not one to be left out of any conversation, milled around, weaving in and out of bare legs. All of a sudden a look of terror came across Uncle Sam's face: he brought his knees together and crossed his arms over his ...mmm.... private parts. Lip glanced down just in time to see Maudie remove her right paw from under Uncle Sam's shorts. Can you believe, Auntie Jennifer. Maudie really has no couth so it is just as well that she becomes royalty. Lip suggested to Uncle Sam that he always wear long pants in our house to avoid a repeat of this embarrassment. If Uncle Sam comes to the door when it is forty below Lip still checks to see if he has long pants on before she lets him in.

I will keep you informed on Maudie's progress into the life of cat royalty. It will not be hard for Maudie but it will be, shall we say, different for Lip and me. For sure.

Love,
Maudie (princess in training)
and Oliver (an accomplished knave)

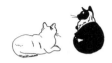

Letter #13 · Books For Birthdays

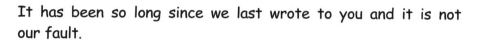

March 22, 2000

Dear Auntie Jennifer:

It has been so long since we last wrote to you and it is not our fault.

Lip has been away gallivanting across the country — who knows where she goes — ignoring us and our needs. It has been dreadful. She is back now and we have told her that it is imperative that she complete her secretarial duties regarding our letters to you TODAY.

This is Maudie speaking.

Lip stayed home with us yesterday and we kept her in bed for a long time. Finally she said she had to get up because Oliver was snoring. We are not sure when this all started but it has become worse over the last few weeks and he sometimes even keeps me awake. I nip him on his knee and he stops. It can be very loud and disconcerting at times. Lip and I are going to have to do something about this.

Lip just had a birthday. She had asked us for a copy of J.R.R. Tolkien's "Lord of the Rings."

We thought that over very seriously and then we decided that that would not be appropriate. It is such a big tome and we know that she would attempt to read it in bed.

Then she would fall asleep and the book would fall, most likely on one or the other of us or both of us and that could cause bodily harm.

We found another book that is much more appropriate. It is called "Cat Massage and much more" by Maryjean Ballner. It is smaller and much easier for Lip to handle. If it does fall it probably would not hurt us. It hasn't fallen yet because it is such a good book that even Lip is enthralled. There are exercises and I have volunteered to be the practice cat. How good this feels, Auntie Jennifer, you have no idea! I will keep Lip on this program and maybe she can get a part-time job as a cat massager. That would be lovely and in the meantime my body will be in great shape. Oliver does not like to be a practice cat as his bones are closer to his skin than mine are. I have a lovely — almost perfect if I do say so myself — thick fur coat that is loose and great to manipulate for massage. I will advise Oliver when I think that Lip is good enough to give him a thorough massage but that won't be for a while yet.

We must close and groom and nap now. We must plan for Saturday's Crewel Stitch-In.

Love,
Oliver and Maudie

Letter #14 • Burns and Crashes

March 31, 2000

Dear Auntie Jennifer:

Well! Did we have a Friday evening last to remember!

This is Oliver speaking.

I was trying desperately to get Lip's attention — she can be so distracted and it is sometimes difficult to get into her face because we are so little. She was fussing in the kitchen and finally, out of frustration, I jumped onto the stove. I knew this move on my part would trigger a reaction as it always had in the past — loud NO NO NO — THAT MIGHT HURT YOU!. YOW! It did. I burned my right paw. Not badly so don't you get alarmed, Auntie Jennifer.

It hurt just enough to understand what that NO NO NO really means. I licked it and it slowly became better. But, I also got lots of attention — hugs and kisses — from Lip. I won't do that again, though. There must be an easier way to get her attention when I have a desperate need for loving. I will have to work on this.

A few minutes later, Maudie fell from the top of the TV to the floor as she was descending from the stereo above the TV. Lip and I were in the dining room discussing my wounds and not paying attention to NO NO NO. We heard this YOW and then a fumble — like a fall coming from the living room. We both knew it was Maudie falling to the floor. Fortunately only her ego — sizeable — was damaged.

Lip used to yell a lot about Maudie and I scaling up to the top of the stereo above the TV.

It is so warm and private up there and we can see and hear almost everything that goes on in the house. She gave up on the yelling some time ago but since Maudie's fall, the yelling is back. Maudie is not very athletic, you know, Auntie Jennifer. She tries to hide this aspect of her nature but I know that she is limited in her jumping skills. She also forgets that she does not have any front nails and this little mental beep sometimes puts her into awkward, physical positions.

The planets were misaligned on Friday night, I tell you. The moon was probably void of course, too.

We understand that you had chemotherapy on Wednesday, the 29th. We pray that this all went well for you and that you are getting better.

Love,
Oliver and Maudie.

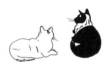

Letter #15 · Wool Candy

April 1, 2000

Dear Auntie Jennifer:

Last Saturday we had the Crewel Stitch-In at our house. This is a great activity and we love to be involved with the planning and the event.

This is Maudie speaking.

Ingrid, Miriam, Cathy and Lip attended for the whole day. Lip put up the card table in the living room and a lot of electrical extension cords appeared from drawers, chairs were repositioned and lamps were strategically placed.

The coffee pot and teapot were always on. Everyone brought their own lunch so we did not have to supervise Lip in lunch preparation duties. Fresh cream appeared for coffee and tea — WE never get this as a treat. Sometimes, when there is no one in the kitchen, we get a chance to lap some up from the cream container. Lip knows what we are doing as she will yell at the precise right moment — "You cats get away from there!" How does she know this? We know that she does not really mean it — this is just a show to make her look good in front of her friends.

But we go along with this anyway. We jump to the floor and scamper upstairs for a few moments and everyone is satisfied.

Only Cathy really likes cats. Ingrid is totally indifferent to us. Miriam seems to be warming to our charms. She has been in our lives since we were babies and we love Auntie Miriam. The other day Oliver jumped up onto the dining room table and Auntie Miriam unconsciously started to hug and stroke him as she listened to Lip. Lip and I could not believe what we were seeing! When Lip abruptly stopped talking Auntie Miriam became aware of what she was doing. She was surprised but you know, I think she liked it. We know that Oliver did but then he has no discrimination when it comes to human hugs and strokes. Anyone will do.

Oliver particularly likes Crewel Stitch-ins as Crewel means Wool and this means candy for Oliver. Oliver could eat all the wool in the world and still want more. Lip is very careful with wool around Oliver — a perpetual struggle for both of them.

Cathy lets Oliver sit on her lap at these stitch-ins. He positions himself on the under side of her work and when the needle comes through the fabric to the wrong side with the wool attached, he tries to bite the wool. For the longest time Cathy could not figure out not only why her wool kept breaking but, how on earth did it become wet? Lip and I knew what was going on but we didn't say anything. We knew she would eventually figure it out, push him to the floor, and that would be the end of Oliver's fun.

After an hour or so, Cathy forgets and Oliver is back in her lap, plotting and planning his next attack on the wool in the needle.

Oliver also plays "hoover." With all this stitching going on, there are pieces of wool dropping onto the floor, sticking to pant legs and chairs. He diligently watches for this and moves very quickly when he sees an opportunity. Sometimes he will grab a whole skein of wool when it accidentally falls to the floor. Great fuss as everyone tries to get it away from him. Oliver is very athletic. I am not athletic, I am voluptuous and beautiful but you know that, Auntie Jennifer.

I sit on the stereo — if Lip will open the cabinet doors — and then I can see and hear everything that goes on. They talk incessantly about everyone who is not here. Gossiping is such fun — I love it!

As you can see this is a great event in our lives — we are still exhausted from Saturday and we have scheduled more and longer naps into our daily routine until we recover from Saturday Crewel Stitch-in.

We hope that your chemotherapy went well and you are recovering.

Love from
Oliver and Maudie.

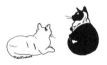

Letter #16 • Mrs. Needy Rustybottoms

April 27, 2000

Dear Auntie Jennifer:

Spring has arrived here and that means the reappearance of Mrs. Needy Rustybottoms.

She is a fair weather cat and only causes havoc in the neighbourhood on nice warm days. She lives across the road from us and we think that she does not like her Lips as she does sly numbers on our Lip whenever she gets the opportunity. As soon as our front door opens here she comes across the parking lot at a busy trot to tell Lip her troubles and woes.

This is Oliver speaking.

We call her Mrs. Needy Rustybottoms because she acts needy in front of Lip. She hugs her legs, rolls on the ground while she tries to convince Lip that life with her would be much more satisfactory than with us. She follows Lip to the garbage dumpster, endlessly chatting about her numerous charms and assets. She is a tabby — very common — but she has rusty bloomers. Probably due to defective genes caused by shady parenting.

If Mrs. Needy Rustybottoms comes up onto our doorstep Maudie goes insane. She screams as if she were instructing pigs on high C notes and flings her body at the screen door. Such a todo! Poor Mrs. Needy Rustybottoms. Although she does not receive any bodily harm from Maudie, her ego and id are temporarily shattered. She slinks away, back to her own doorstep with her ears sagging from verbal assault, her tail dragging behind her.

Maudie has just learned that kickboxing lessons might assist in her efforts to ward off the threat of Mrs. Needy Rustybottoms moving in with us. She has been diligently trying to convince Lip that kickboxing lessons for Siamese cats would vastly improve our lot in life. Lip advised Maudie that her verbal missiles are more than adequate to fend off any threat by Mrs. Needy Rustybottoms.

At least Mrs. Needy Rustybottoms is smart enough to know a good home when she sees one.

Lip advised us that you had your fifth chemotherapy yesterday. We hope it was not too painful and you are feeling better today.

We had Lip send you flowers from us yesterday. We took money from our allowance savings for this. I contributed more than Maudie did as she has had several penalties lately for incorrect behaviour.

Love,
Oliver and Maudie.

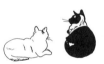

Letter #17 · Midnight Pizza

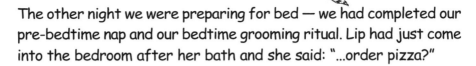

May 11, 2000

Dear Auntie Jennifer:

The other night we were preparing for bed — we had completed our pre-bedtime nap and our bedtime grooming ritual. Lip had just come into the bedroom after her bath and she said: "...order pizza?"

This is Oliver speaking.

She wanted us to order pizza? Well! We had never done this before! How on earth do we do that? Maudie said "I think that we do this on the downstairs phone."

We went downstairs and pondered and planned how we were going to complete this assigned task. Lip did not tell us what she wanted on the pizza so we assumed that the choices were for us to decide. After much thought and discussion we agreed on a sardine pizza with no tomatoes and green pepper. Green pepper sounds like something that would not benefit our digestive systems and could cause harm.

After great fumbling and screeching at the phone order man we managed to order the pizza. This took most of the night for us to do this. And Lip wonders why we sleep most of the day!

The pizza man finally arrived at 4:30 am. We were so exhausted from all of this we just let him bang on the door. We knew that Lip would finally hear him and she could come down and pay him. We don't handle money matters.

Well! Was Lip upset over this! "Who ordered this pizza at this hour? You will both be punished for this!"

Go figure. After the dust settled it seems we misunderstood what Lip said in the beginning. She says she said "I smell pizza. I wonder who ordered pizza?"

We are going to pay more attention to what Lip says from now on or we could land in REAL TROUBLE.

We hope that you are feeling well Auntie Jennifer. We will meditate for you when you have your last chemotherapy treatment. We are looking forward to your last treatment, too.

Love,
Maudie and Oliver

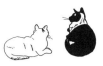

Letter #18 · Fur Ball Sale

June 1, 2000

Dear Auntie Jennifer:

Last weekend all of the people in this area had a garage sale. But it wasn't really a garage sale because there are no garages around here. It was actually a parking lot sale. The sale was very successful by all accounts, so Lip tells us. (We are indoor cats so we only know what goes on from what we can see from our bench in the dining room window.)

This is Oliver speaking.

Mrs. Needy Rustybottoms managed to get into everyone's way and face during the sale.

Several people were not pleased with her behaviour. But, she did come up with a great idea:

A CAT GARAGE SALE!

Maudie and I think this is a grand idea and can not believe that we did not think of it for ourselves. Imagine! Mrs. Needy Rustybottoms being so clever.

Maudie suggested that I go through all of the toys to see what we could sell. Well, Auntie Jennifer, I don't want to sell any of our toys. I told Maudie this and she said "Do it, Oliver or I will sell them all ! Or worse, I will give them away!" I get very nervous when Maudie speaks to me like this, Auntie Jennifer, and I have to sit down and scratch or bite my nails until my nerves realign. But, I did go through the toys and I came up with seven:

A rope tied in a knot, an old sock, four wind-up mice (broken wind-up mice), and a plastic ball that used to have a bell in it. (We think that Lip removed the bell as we have no idea how the bell disappeared).

I suggested to Maudie that she could sort through all of her combs and brushes and perhaps sell some of them at the Cat Garage Sale. She said, "NO WAY OLIVER! SMARTEN UP!" (Time out for a scratch).

We have found other items for the sale: furballs (a dime a dozen for those), used cat food tins, kitty litter bags, shredded furniture, chewed wool (I have a lot of this hidden around the house), ratty towels that once lined our basket, broken vases, snarled embroidery thread, punctured bridge cards and a whole big bag of dust bunnies! Lip contributed the dust bunnies.

We asked Lip if she had any suggestions of items that we could sell at our sale. She said our cat fridge magnets might be a good idea. No way! We have one from Ron Robinson for his Radio

Weekend show and we would never part with that. It is actually on the stove, Auntie Jennifer, right beside our food station. We look at it every day.

We have no idea what Mrs. Needy Rustybottoms has for sale but we don't think she will have much.

Maudie has decided that she will be the hostess cat and greet all our customers as she has the most charm and beauty (so she says). Mrs. Needy Rustybottoms, who is actually quite good looking, will tidy and keep the area clean (a gofer) and I will handle all the accounts of trade and negotiation. High quality cat treats and food will be the preferred method of payment.

We expect all our neighbours will come to this grand event.

There is Black Bart. He is a rogue and he has his eye on Maudie. He is very gallant and charming but he does not pay much attention to his person. He has patches of fur missing due to battles of the night and one ear droops significantly. Maudie will have an opportunity to put on her royal airs for Black Bart. He will fall to the ground, smitten by her charms!

Mickey, Ben and Casey live with Suzanne (who is very nice and very pretty). They will come all as a family. Lip bought stuff from Suzanne at the adult garage sale that was not really a garage sale so we are sure that Mickey, Ben and Casey will buy some of our high quality items. Ben and Casey are both orange marmalade and they look like each other. They too, are indoor cats so Suzanne will have to escort them to the sale. We have heard via the feline grapevine that Mickey is somewhat "light fingered" so we will assign Mrs. Needy Rustybottoms to watch him carefully. If we catch him lifting items we will have Maudie deal with him. Need I say more!

We have invited Sally Sue who used to live with Uncle Sam and Auntie Betty. Sally Sue does not like us. She knew us when we were babies and we drove her to distraction and she has become quite weird. She will probably decline due to other engagements.

Mineux is all white and getting on in years. He has a bad temperament. We invited him because Jenette lives with him and she takes very good care of us when Lip is away.

We know that he will barter with us and try to get really good deals.

Jasmin and Astee will also come. Astee is very shy and he will hang on to Jasmin while he is at the sale. Lip talks to Astee all the time out the kitchen window as he sits at his screen door.

We must sign off now Auntie Jennifer, as you can see we have a lot of work to do to prepare for our GARAGE SALE TO DIE FOR!

We hope that your last Chemotherapy treatment is nice and easy.

Love
Maudie and Oliver.

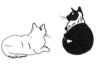

Letter #19 · Summer Jobs

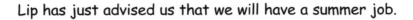

June 6, 2000

Dear Auntie Jennifer:

Lip has just advised us that we will have a summer job.

CAN YOU BELIEVE!

This is Maudie speaking.

Yesterday a spider was found on the staircase. He was doing no harm but Lip freaked out, scared him, and set us spinning into motion.

We are now to control all the other livestock — small stuff — in the house. Lip wants to see no more of this and we are to deal with it.

We find all of the small stuff that comes into the house in the summer very amusing and entertaining. Oliver bats them around as if he were playing hockey for one of the major teams. Lip should look into getting him on one of the teams. I understand that some of the players are really retarded in the talent field. Then we would be rich, rich, rich!

Sometimes they get under the fridge and probably die a slow torturous death. I think I will get the cleaning ladies to move the fridge the next time they are here. This is really all I am willing to contribute to this summer employment nonsense. Oliver can take care of the rest. Work like this could interfere with my grooming schedule which is very heavy in the summer.

Several male cats come up to the patio door windows on nice summer days to drool over my fantastic beauty and I have no intention of letting my admiring fans down.

Four more cats are coming to our garage sale, Auntie Jennifer — "April" and "Amanda," two spinster cats who live with Brenda. They don't get out much so they will have a good time. "Shmoo" and "Nebbie" live with Barry and Andrea. We don't know much about them but we understand that they are coming on bikes — can you imagine!

Must prepare for nap #3,

Love from
Maudie and Oliver

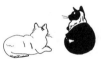

Letter #20 · Visit To Dr. Peter

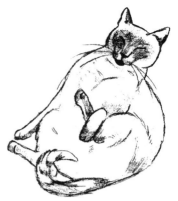

June 21, 2000

Dear Auntie Jennifer:

On Monday we had our annual check-ups.

This is Oliver speaking.

We have no warning that we are going to Dr. Peter's for our check-up and shots.

Lip is very smooth and sneaky about getting us into our carriers for this journey.

She goes down the basement stairs — we always go with her into the basement. It is dark and dingy down there so we must protect her from ghosts and shadows that move on the fringe of our vision. She calmly walks by our carriers and as we are following very closely to provide escort she has an opportunity to grab us and stuff us — yes! Stuff us into our carriers! Maudie got to the top of the stairs but Lip caught up to her, she stopped to look back and that was her fate!

We go in the car. Only one of us can ride in the front seat — that is the best place — so we take turns. Whoever rides in the front going to must ride in the back coming from. This was quite uneventful as it was not rush hour so Lip did not have great opportunities to jump on the brakes and scare us witless.

We were greeted by the two Bettys. They both love us and are very kind. They love to cuddle me as I am a great lover of people who wear skirts. Four cats live at Dr. Peter's place — Toes (he has seven toes on his front feet, sometimes called Toey), Max (no tail, don' t know how this happened), Thomas (the most senior cat. He has a part-time job at the police station down the way- we don't know what he does there) and Wiseman (named after the dentist who has an office next door.).

Hanging from the ceiling is a large bird cage — just out of reach. Toes was in great trouble today as a bird had gone missing overnight and he was suspected of this heinous crime. He looked like he was not suffering much from this as he was napping on the check-in counter. Even as he napped, he had a smirk on his face.

Wiseman has the hots for Maudie.

Betty K weighed us and they were all pleased that we had maintained our perfect weight.

Peter then poked and prodded us — this puts us in very undignified configurations. We do not like this at all. Then we both were poked with a sharp needle. This should not happen to cats, Auntie Jennifer. It scared me so much that I leaped from the table right back into my carrier.

Needless to say, a very stressful day for us.

It will take some intense grooming and deep naps to recover and return to normal after this awesome experience.

Lip tells us Auntie Jennifer, that you have started on your radiation treatments and are still working. This is lovely and we will pray for you.

Love,
Maudie and Oliver

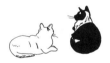

Letter #21 · Oliver Abandoned

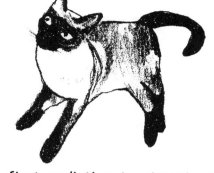

June 22, 2000

Dear Auntie Jennifer:

Lip told us that you had your first radiation treatment on Wednesday. We hope and pray that it went well and that it did what it was supposed to do.

On Monday, Maudie went into the hospital to have some dental surgery. She was gone all day and I was abandoned.

This is Oliver speaking.

Sunday night Lip took our food away from us. I did not understand this as it has never, ever happened before. It was just gone! I was starving throughout the night and was forced to nibble on the palm tree in the living room. This is not really satisfactory as it makes me spit up. But at least it keeps my pipes clean.

Then, first thing in the morning Maudie is quickly put into her cat carrier, the food dish — full of food — is returned to its place and I am left all alone. I did not like this at all, Auntie Jennifer. I prefer the company of others rather than my own.

I had a big feast, intense scrub up and then a short nap. Just not the same without Maudie. So, I decided that I must make the best of this horrible situation. I started by taking all the toys up to the bed, This took quite a while as there are several toys and I had to find them all. I was exhausted so I had a longer than usual nap with all the toys around me. Small comfort but not the same. I sat on the love seat and looked forlornly out of the window, contemplating my fate. Mrs. Needy Rustybottoms appeared and strolled through Lip's Zen garden, knocking the roof off the little temple. She has no grace, Auntie Jennifer, none at all. But, if I could have, I would have let her in. She was better than nothing.

Late in the day Lip and Maudie returned. Well, I think it was Maudie. She looked like Maudie, sounded like Maudie, and walked like Maudie. But she did not smell like Maudie. I was so confused about this. Is this a pretend Maudie? Did something happen to the real Maudie?

I hissed at her and this really upset Lip and "Maudie." Then I was really confused, Auntie Jennifer. Everyone kept their distance for a few days and I did not hiss anymore. I have never hissed before and I did not want to upset Lip and "Maudie."

After a few days I realized that it was the real Maudie. She just came back with a bad smell on her. She now smells like my Maudie and I am so pleased.

Maudie is supposed to take some pills but after the second (of fourteen) Lip has abandoned this exercise. It is summer and the windows are open. One of the neighbours was so startled by the noise coming from the kitchen window she knocked on the door to see if someone was in pain. Lip replied, "Not yet."

Everything is now back to normal, Auntie Jennifer. Maudie is her usual royal self and all is right with my world!

Love,
Oliver and Maudie

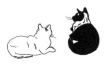

Letter #22 · Kitty Litter Chaos

July 11, 2000

Dear Auntie Jennifer:

It was a dark and stormy night — until the lightning started.

This is Maudie speaking.

Last Thursday night Lip finally returned home from all her gallivanting around.

She said that she saw you and that you looked wonderful. She can gallivant all she likes for that good news! Although, Auntie Jennifer, she did assure me that I am still prettier than you.

We all went to bed very early after we helped Lip unpack and return the suitcase to the basement. Only when the suitcase is returned to its space in the basement can we relax.

But, in the meantime, Oliver started bringing his toys upstairs. I should have twigged to that. He sensed trouble!

The lightning woke us about two a.m. and it was so bright that we thought Lip would get out her book and start to read to us. We couldn't sleep so reading was in order. Then the thunder started so we would not have been able to hear Lip reading to us anyway...

(A good mystery is what we are presently involved with so it would have been very appropriate.)

Shortly after the thunder started, the rains came. It poured dogs for hours, Auntie Jennifer. No cat with any smarts would have been caught out there, let me tell you!

We all got up at seven in the morning and it was still pouring dogs. We sensed that rather than stay in bed as we usually try to do, we should get up to see how things were doing.

Things were not doing well at all! The basement floor was wet and we were not able to get to our litter boxes without getting our paws wet. This was an awful situation! Oliver had accompanied Lip downstairs to see the damage (I knew that all that damp would not be good for my fur so I stayed upstairs where it was dry and warm.)

Lip tried to convince Oliver that it was not really that wet and that it would start to dry and we should have no trouble navigating to our litter box. No trouble indeed! Oliver took a very firm stance on this matter and would not allow Lip to leave things as they were. Finally, she got the message and moved our litter boxes over to the bottom of the stairs so that we would not have to cross the wet floor.

When Lip came home from work she cleaned a path to where our litter boxes are suppose to be. That was satisfactory.

Nasty business these prairie summer thunderstorms, Auntie Jennifer. I hope you do not experience the same.

We are so pleased to hear that you are looking well and feeling well.

Love,
Maudie and Oliver

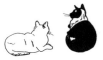

Letter #23 • Rat Patrol

July 20, 2000

Dear Auntie Jennifer:

A day to celebrate! Your last radiation treatment and we are so pleased with this. We have plans for a little celebration this evening — just the three of us. We will have instructions for Lip on this when she gets home.

Now, on to very shocking business, Auntie Jennifer. Lip tells us that you have rats -yes rats! three of them! — in your office. We cannot imagine how this came about. We are stunned to paralyzation with this information.

Lip tells us that the reason you have rats in your office is because your office is so messy. We know that Lip does not always tell us the truth so we are not going to buy into this story about your messy office.

But, we must help you rid your office of these rats. This will just not do!

This is Maudie speaking.

We have no experience with rats — we only have on-the-job-experience with little things like spiders, ants, mosquitoes, etc.

Actually, Oliver has the on-the-job experience. This summer job business is frightfully boring, if you want my opinion. So when these little critters surface I convince Oliver that it is to his benefit to develop this skill because he is better than I at this mundane task.

We have a plan though, to rid your office of the rats. Hang in, there, Auntie Jennifer!

The first part of the plan is we send Lip to the book store to find a book or books on rat riddance from offices. We will study this — with Lip's help — and then when we are expert and have a plan, we will come to your office to save you from the rats.

I suggested to Oliver that maybe we should get Black Bart, one of my suitors, in on this. Although we have never talked about rat control, I am sure that this is a subject that Black Bart would know a lot about.

The second part of the plan is to have Lip book three first class seats -we are Siamese after all — to come to your office. We will probably have to clean Black Bart up a bit to get him into first class but with my knowledge and grooming techniques, this should not be a problem. He can also be in charge of my carry-on baggage. I will have to take my combs and brushes with me and we will probably need some weapons for the rat raid.

Lip tells us that we may have a problem with our weapons and security. I am sure with my charm and beauty I will be able to convince the security people of this urgent need to get our equipment to your office. Lip is also going to see if she can have us preboarded. That would be nice, before the human stampede starts — all that shoving and pushing and being uppity to the flight attendants.

We understand that we can order special meals — delightful! We will treat Black Bart to shrimp and crabmeat and of course, salmon. Oliver thinks we should go easy on the special meal for Black Bart as he may not be accustomed to all this rich food and he may have a spit up in-flight. Oliver and I would find that very embarrassing. Lip tells us that there will be a sandbox for us under our seats, beside my carry-on baggage.

There is no need for you to meet us at the airport, Auntie Jennifer. We will conduct the rat raid in the still of the night when they are probably asleep and least expect us. We can work in the dark, that is not a problem.

One day soon, when you come to work, you will find absolutely no rats. We won't leave one trace of them! You won't even know we were there!

Love,
Oliver and Maudie

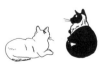

Letter #24 · Your Visit To Us

December 12, 2000

Dear Auntie Jennifer:

We want you to know how much we enjoyed your visit last week.

This is Oliver speaking.

I thought that you looked absolutely fabulous, Auntie Jennifer, and Maudie said that you looked ...ok. She is a bit jealous, I think, when other good-looking females come into the house and challenge her charm, voluptuousness, and beauty.

Which you did, indeed!

She would like me to tell you that she thanks you so much for rescuing her from the snowbank. She did not realize how cold it was and she does not understand why the snow on the lawn is not removed prior to her short sorties outside in the winter. She always gives her pig screech just before she comes back into the house. It is nothing you did. She likes to alert the neighbours that she is being held hostage and being abused.

I enjoyed my pre-bedtime nap on your lap — for three hours! YOW! I never have that on Lip's lap. I get poked with knitting needles, she squirms, drops stitches that I have to retrieve from the floor — up and down, up and down.

She answers the phone, switches TV channels, scratches, sneezes, drinks coffee and wine and carries on like you would not believe. Your lap is much better for extended, required naps.

It is very cold here and we run away from the front door when we suspect that it might be opened. Why Lip would want to go out in weather like this is beyond us. She has placed our basket on top of a heat vent in the closet upstairs. It is very comfortable and we get to watch everyone who comes into the bathroom, which is a bonus full of all kinds of surprises.

I must sign off now and listen to Maudie's latest opus on her new opera. She said that if I listen and give CONSTRUCTIVE criticism, she will clean my ears for me.

Love,
Oliver and Maudie

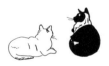

Letter #25 • She Who Hisses
The Loudest Is To Be Obeyed

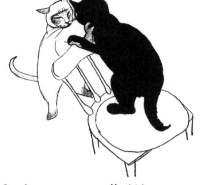

October 17, 2001

Dear Auntie Jennifer:

Lip has told us that you are not feeling very well. We are so very sorry to hear this and we will meditate for your quick return to health.

We have been in serious trouble for the last two nights. Lip has been so upset with us that she told us this morning that if our night-time behaviour does not improve NOW we will have to find alternate sleeping arrangements.

We do not want that. We like sleeping with Lip as she produces lots of warmth for our comfort. She turns the heat way down at night so she is the only source of additional heat available to us at night, so we must address this situation.

This is Maudie speaking.

All of these night-time behaviour problems are not my fault although Oliver will tell you otherwise.

It all started on Saturday night when we had Rumoli at our house. This is a monthly event for Lip. It only happens at our house every third month but it is always great excitement and noise. We participate in this by making sure we are impeccably groomed, charming and intensely interested in all goings on.

Oliver was in his element with five humans in the seated position. He makes a pest of himself by travelling from lap to lap to lap to lap.

I challenged Oliver to go around the table to every lap without touching the floor. This of course involved some travel on the table and the buffet. This was very stressful because he knew that if he knocked the pennies or the chips off the table he would be yelled at and sent to his room. Oliver has intense concentration and, lo, indeed he did it, Auntie Jennifer! He even went back to Auntie Betty's lap and Lip's lap several times. But, that was easy as they were sitting beside one another and he knew he was always welcome there.

And, here is the problem, Auntie Jennifer. Because Oliver received a lot of hugs and kisses from five humans all wearing different perfumes (Yes! Even the men, can you believe!) he smells gross! Gross! So, every time he comes near me, I hiss at him and give him a swat to go away. This wakes up Lip and she hisses and swats. We all reposition and try and get back to sleep. Then Oliver starts to crawl over to me and here we go again!

She who hisses the loudest must be obeyed! We must get our act together.

I have offered to help Oliver clean himself of this horrid smell. It is important that we keep the status quo, as winter is coming on.

Love,
Oliver and Maudie

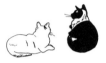

Letter #26 · Our Winter Outing

December 3, 2001

Dear Auntie Jennifer:

Lip has told us that you are very sick again. We are very, very, sorry to hear this. We will pray for you every day and you are in our thoughts constantly.

You must rest and don't worry about things. Things don't matter. Short naps are good too. Whenever we feel peaked we do a wee wash and a short nap. You must drink lots of water too, Auntie Jennifer. It flushes out your system.

We had our annual winter outing last Friday night.

This is Oliver speaking.

We are indoor cats and really don't have much interest in going outside. Well, I don't but sometimes Maudie has the urge. She tells me that things are not right out there and she could sort out the world in no time flat. Of course, Lip won't allow this. That would just cause a whole bunch of other problems for Lip.

But, we really love to go out in the first snowfall. So Lip allows this for a few moments. I always stay to the swept sidewalk and only go a few yards from the front door. Then I come back in, always before Maudie. She can stay out longer than I can as my bones are closer to the skin than Maudie's are. She has more protection from the elements, so to speak.

Maudie stayed out for a long time. I was frantic because I could not see her so I raced from the dining room window to the kitchen window to the front door and back again. I could not see her! Lip said she will come back, don't worry, she won't go far without her grooming tools. Finally, I think that Lip became concerned. She started to put her boots on.

Just as Lip was getting ready to go out the door to find Maudie the most horrid sound rattled both of us.

"MMMMRRAAAACCCCKK!!!!"

One of our neighbours was coming out of her door and dropped her garbage on the doorstep. "What the hell was that?" she said.

That, was Maudie, displaying her displeasure at meeting a closed door. I was elated, she had returned!

Lip let her in and said, "Maudie, we are going to send you for elocution lessons. You look like a cat, act like a cat, have an exceptional cat attitude, but you just don't sound like a cat."

"Whatever," said Maudie, as she inspected her nails.

Please take care of yourself, Auntie Jennifer.

Love,
Oliver and Maudie

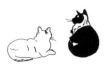

Letter #27 • Mrs. Perkins' Visit

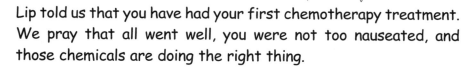

December 19, 2001

Dear Auntie Jennifer:

Lip told us that you have had your first chemotherapy treatment. We pray that all went well, you were not too nauseated, and those chemicals are doing the right thing.

This is Maudie speaking.

We had a visitor this fall. Mrs Perkins. She is the President of Embroiderers' Association of Canada. Lip is a lowly member of this organization so having the President stay with us was such an honour. She was billeted — we don't know what that means — with us for three days.

There was great excitement and activity to prepare for Mrs. Perkins' arrival. Lip scrubbed everything in sight, including us, cooked and baked wonderful things. This was the most activity we have seen around here in a long time.

Mrs. Perkins arrived on Friday afternoon. We were introduced to her and she commented on my extraordinary beauty and Oliver's elegant manners. We were prepared to be on our very best behaviour.

Tea was served. We stayed off the dining room table for this. Lip said that we could sit on chairs but we would not receive any servings from the table. This is new but we thought that we would go along with this to impress Mrs. Perkins as that is obviously what Lip was striving to do.

After tea, Mrs. Perkins took her bags upstairs and unpacked in the den. We tried to assist her — we know a lot about packing and unpacking suitcases — but she graciously declined our assistance.

After dinner, Lip took Mrs. Perkins somewhere, came home to read the new temporary rules to us, then collected Mrs. Perkins. Now it is bedtime.

We tried to assist with the bed making — we know a lot about bed making and we think that Martha Stewart has it all wrong. Again, our assistance was thwarted.

Lo, Mrs. Perkins shut her bedroom door for the night. Well! This is very new. We don't have closed doors in our house. Sometimes a person will close the bathroom door but we know that that is only temporary and that is okay. But a bedroom door shut for the whole night is not acceptable.

We were prepared to sleep with Mrs. Perkins and it is obvious Lip did not tell her what a joy having our company in bed really is. Oliver was devastated. He whined and scratched at the door for hours. Lip did nothing as she knew that it would not help. After about four hours of this, Oliver came to bed with Lip and me. He was exhausted and totally stressed.

The next day Lip drove Mrs. Perkins to her meetings after breakfast and Lip returned and started on some really serious cooking and baking. Although the house smelled wonderful we were very much neglected.

Mrs. Perkins returned and she and Lip prepared to go to a potluck supper.

Lip had almost finished cleaning up the kitchen — a few pots and pans were in the sink in hot soapy water.

Then. Disaster struck!!!

As you know, Auntie Jennifer, our cat grass grows on the window sill above the kitchen sink. This is the only place in the house that it will grow so we have limited access- Lip thinks it is limited — to the kitchen counter to get to the shelf with our grass. It is very important for our diet that we eat our grass regularly. I think that Oliver eats more grass than food as he is always up there.

Because of the closed door and neglect Oliver really was stressed out. As Lip, Mrs. Perkins and I were sitting at the dining room table chatting, Oliver was at the grass pot. Then, he threw up into the kitchen sink.

Major, major embarrassment!

I jumped from my chair and disappeared to a secret place and Mrs. Perkins ran up the stairs. Lip was heard to say "Oh, Oliver..." Lip cleaned up Oliver's mess and Mrs. Perkins returned and said. "It happens in the best of families." It does?

Oliver was more embarrassed than Lip was. I returned to my chair and started major work on my nails — like nothing had happened. Oliver retired to the basket upstairs.

Shortly after Lip and Mrs. Perkins went out to the potluck supper. Lip told Ingrid the story and she is still laughing.

We don't have many overnight visitors, Auntie Jennifer, so we must have a board meeting with Lip to set up a few ground rules for these occasions. After all, this is our house too.

We are praying for you Auntie Jennifer. Get lots of rest and eat healthy things.

Maybe not grass.

Love,
Oliver and Maudie

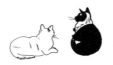

Letter #28 · Nods and Naps

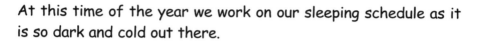

December 28, 2001

Dear Auntie Jennifer:

At this time of the year we work on our sleeping schedule as it is so dark and cold out there.

We have had to explain to Lip that sleep is not necessarily sleep to us. So, we will give you a short lesson too, Auntie Jennifer, on this subject.

This is Maudie speaking.

There are four categories of "sleep" as we know it. They are:
nods
naps
lap naps
deep sleeps (industrial strength).

1. Nods

    These are best conducted in quiet, warm sunlight, preferably after a light meal and major scrub. The armrest of the loveseat or the window seat in the dining room are the best places in this house for that. Nods allows the eyes to be closed but the head cannot be touching any object; it must remain upright. We are semi-aware of what is going on around us — Lip dropping things in the kitchen — but we do not react.

2. Naps

Naps allow us to get into very comfortable positions and the head can be resting on the surface. I like to take my naps on top of the TV. When it is on it provides great warmth. It is also is a safe place. Well, once, I was too comfortable and I tumbled to the floor. Great loss of dignity when that happened, Auntie Jennifer. We have to be yelled at or otherwise displaced to get us out of a true nap mode. We spend a lot of time napping.

3. Lap naps

This is an Oliver speciality. As soon as Lip sits down, he is right there, scrambling to get onto her lap. He will spend hours on her lap when he gets the opportunity. She stretches out her legs onto the stool and he curls into the lap nap mode. She moves and reaches, squirms, pokes him with knitting needles, drops the remote control on his head, spills wine or coffee on his tail but he just lap naps on. Then, Lip will suddenly stand and there is Oliver, clinging to her legs or the chair, in a state of shock, jarred into consciousness. I wonder about Oliver's level of intelligence sometimes.

4. Deep Sleeps

This is the best of all. Our basket in the closet is placed over a hot air vent and we spend most of the day here when Lip is not home and we have no need to supervise her actions. We are in the true prone position, curled up together. Sometimes, Uncle Sam comes over and we don't even know he was here! We wake when it is time for Lip to come home. It is important that we greet her at the door so we set our internal alarm clocks for her arrival. Sometimes, Oliver will get carried away with his snoring and I have to poke him. He shifts, and all is well again.

There, Auntie Jennifer! Now you know all about nods and naps.

We are praying for you and we hope you are warm and comfortable. Nods and Naps are good for humans too so we hope you will try them.

Love,
Oliver and Maudie

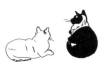

Letter #29 · Hal The Computer

January 15, 2002

Dear Auntie Jennifer:

We understand that you had a chemotherapy treatment on the 9th. We are very late writing to you but it is not our fault.

We have a new computer and Lip is still learning how to use it.

We are not sure what this is all about but it certainly has added excitement to our lives. The computer is ugly — black and squat and it sits on the desk in the den, doing what appears as nothing. It does purr, but not like we purr. More like how the refrigerator purrs. Both sound quite offensive. We have the furnace, the refrigerator, now the computer. What next?

This is Oliver speaking.

Maudie is a great purrer — diva quality. She can't sing but she can purr. I am trying to convince her to give diva purring lessons to the refrigerator and the computer. She says that they don't really have the basic talent to learn what she has to teach. A waste of her valuable time.

The other night Lip was working away at the computer and it was getting very close to normal bedtime. I was having a pre-bedtime nap and Maudie was working on a nod on the chesterfield in the den.

Lip was finishing up her e-mail and was using spell check.

This is a good thing because Lip is not well known for her spelling skills. Lip was putting this to good use and spell check came across some bad words that Lip had typed. Frequently, Lip uses bad words. We cover our ears when that happens to let her know that we do not approve of this behaviour. The words that she used were — oh, we cannot say what she used but, Auntie Jennifer, it was something like this: son of a female dog. That, of course, to us is the lowest of life forms. Spell check flashed a message to Lip that said (sic) "This is a sexist remark. Would you like to change it?"

Lip shrieked — yes shrieked, Auntie Jennifer! We were startled out of our wits! "Big brother is alive and well!" shouted Lip. That's nice. She immediately shut the computer down, turned to us and said "Bedtime. Now!" We shuffled down the hall after Lip as going to bed seemed to be the right thing to do.

Maybe the computer is not such a bad thing if it encourages Lip to clean up her act. We would like that and would look more kindly on that ugly black thing.

The next morning Lip announced that the computer now has a name: "HAL."

We hope that you are getting good naps, nods and sleeps and lots of rest and good food. We are praying for you, Auntie Jennifer.

Love,
Oliver and Maudie

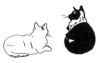

Letter #30 · Rules for Retirement

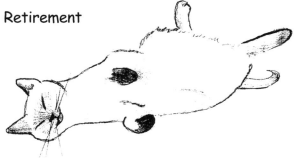

January 29, 2002

Dear Auntie Jennifer:

A few days ago Lip announced to us at dinner time that she would be retiring in the very near future.

We had no idea what "retirement" meant so we had Lip explain it to us in enough detail so that we could comprehend.

This is Maudie speaking.

Oliver and I had a conference on this as it was clear that this "retirement" business would have a profound impact on our daily routine. It became clear that we would have to draft some rules of retirement to protect our very comfortable lifestyle. We worked for days on this, Auntie Jennifer, and we think that we were most fair to all concerned, considering.

Here are the rules as we presented them to Lip:

1. There will be no more mornings
    Five days a week the radio turns itself on, Lip jumps out of bed, jarring us out of position and into consciousness. Then, we are pushed off the bed so that it can be made. Imagine! We know that Martha Stewart is responsible for this. It is

dark, cold and why humans want to move around at this time of the night is beyond us. If Lip wants to do mornings she must give us two days notice so that we are not disturbed and can maintain our sleep pattern — in our basket or on the chesterfield in the den.

2. New Grooming Schedule and Services
   Now that Lip has more time on her hands, we expect daily brushings for no less than five minutes. Massages — from the book- will be scheduled for no less than twice a week, and on demand. Oliver will have his nails done at least once a week and more, if required. I will continue to do my own nails but I will now schedule lap time for this.

3. Litter Box Protocol
   We have accepted in the past that our litter box is attended to once a day. Lip was working and we realized that she did her best, under the circumstances. Now we feel that three times a day would be more appropriate.

4. More Bingo, less Bridge
   As Lip will have a reduced income, we feel she should put her leisure time to activities that produce extra money. This is for the well-being of us all. Bridge does not have any monetary rewards. Bingo does have potential for financial gain and Lip should reduce her time spent at the bridge table — it is only frustrating to her anyway, Auntie Jennifer — and spend more time pursuing dollars for us.

5. Reading

   When we were babies, Lip use to read out loud to us. She would sit on the floor in the den with her legs stretched out, we would climb into her lap and curl up together like yin and yang. We got as far as page eleven of "David Copperfield." We would eventually nod off but we really liked that. It is now time to finish "David Copperfield."

6. Afternoon Naps

   This is mandatory. What else can I say?

7. More Board Meetings

   When Lip works, she is totally frazzled. She never listens to us.

   When we do get her attention she says that she can hear us but she is not listening. For sure.

   And we tell her important things, Auntie Jennifer! Things like — there is a spider crossing the basement floor. There is a full moon rising. Robert Rabbit is peeing in the garden.

   We expect more structured board meetings and Lip is now expected to pay more attention.

8. More CBC FM

   We will have quiet time between three and six every weekday afternoon and listen to Jurgen Gothe. Lip may knit or do needlework at this time but she cannot make noise — too soon after our afternoon naps. We like Jurgen Gothe because he talks cat talk.

We presented these rules to Lip yesterday in our most business-like manner.

She thought for a long while on this. Finally, she stood up, put on her coat and announced: "I'm going out for a while — to find a job."

We hope your treatment today, Auntie Jennifer, is working wonders in your body and we are praying for you.

Love,
Oliver and Maudie

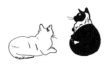

Letter #31 · Our Valentine

February 14, 2002

Dear Auntie Jennifer:

Would you be our Valentine?

This is Oliver speaking.

We would be most honoured.

Love,
Oliver and Maudie

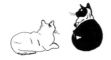

Letter #32 • More Hal Business

February 14, 2002

Dear Auntie Jennifer:

HAL the computer has been living with us for some time now. We have not yet got a full read on him, but we are working on it.

This is Maudie speaking.

We find that he is really quite boring — until Lip starts to push his buttons. Then an interaction between Lip and HAL starts that is really quite x-rated, Auntie Jennifer. We are going to have to remind Lip to close the windows when the weather gets warmer. The neighbours would not approve.

We call this Lip-HAL computer speak — quite different than normal computer speak. We do not understand it at all but we know that HAL is also pushing Lip's buttons. Lip speaks in a tongue very foreign to us. It is like this, Auntie Jennifer:

&^&()^&^^$#??//&^!!!!

HAL says nothing — just purrs along.

HAL comes with his own mouse. Imagine! This mouse is not like any known to us. First of all, he has no fur. He is very bald and we can't seem to get our teeth into him. He is about as boring as HAL as he shows no fear of us. That is not mouse-like. He has the longest tail we have ever seen. HAL sits on it. We have tried to drag the mouse away from HAL but HAL will not let go. Control freak.

One day, Lip came home and found the mouse hanging by his tail from the desk — still HAL would not let go.

We were ...um, "spoken to" about that.

The mouse now has his own bed. That is weird also. Very flat and not nest-like at all, but he seems content enough with this arrangement. He really is dumb, dumb, big time.

We are not sure but we sometimes think we hear another cat when Lip and HAL are having a go at each other's egos.

We will keep you posted on this last finding, Auntie Jennifer.

Lip said that you are not feeling very well and are having some more chemotherapy. We will pray for you, Auntie Jennifer that the chemicals will work this time.

Love,
Oliver and Maudie

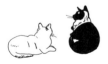

Letter #33 · Feng Shui

February 28, 2002

Dear Auntie Jennifer:

Last night we had a board meeting. Lip explained to us the basics — as she knows them — of feng shui and announced that we were going to start living our lives accordingly.

This is Maudie speaking.

We found this meeting very boring. Lip went on and on about ancient Chinese numerical systems, twelve earthly branches, ten heavenly systems and how we need sheng chi, not si chi in our lives. I did my nails and Oliver cleaned the base of his tail.

The next step was to find the qi centre of every room. This is the most sensitive area in a room. We know this instinctively and one of us would just sit down in the qi centre but Lip just didn't get it. She had a tape measure and fussed and carried on for hours.

Next step was to find the yin and yang area of each room. We know about these places too and tried to show her this by playing in the yang spots and being pensive in the yin spots. Went right over her head, Auntie Jennifer. She really does not pay attention.

It was announced that in the next few days we will be conducting a major clean up of the basement and the closets will be purged.

Cleaning the basement is very stressful for us — causes great dust-ups, relocation of stuff, and noise. We think that the closets are just fine but here we go again!

Lip stated that there will be no more clutter. Clutter causes bad chi and we can't have that. We love clutter, Auntie Jennifer. Clutter is a major cat thing. And we don't see any bad chi with clutter.

According to the books that Lip has on feng shui, the bed must be relocated. We have not done this yet but it is just a matter of time.

As you can see, our lives with Lip are not always easy. We do love her but at times she drives us to distraction.

We noticed that Lip has a book on feng shui in the garden. We will have to warn Robert Rabbit about the upset he is going to have this coming summer.

Please take good care of yourself, Auntie Jennifer. We are all praying for you everyday to get better so that you can come and see us. Have lots of naps and eat healthy.

Love,
Oliver and Maudie

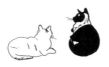

Letter #34 · The Green Plaid Chair

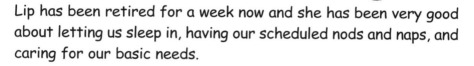

March 25, 2002

Dear Auntie Jennifer:

Lip has been retired for a week now and she has been very good about letting us sleep in, having our scheduled nods and naps, and caring for our basic needs.

But, we are having a problem with our green plaid wing chair.

This is Oliver speaking.

For as long as we can remember, this has been our chair. It was made for us, we are sure. We have had parties with about fourteen people in the living room and we have never been asked to give the chair up to a human being. Lip's friends understand that the chair is ours.

Maudie and I fit into the chair perfectly. It has three sides to support us and protect us from spirits, unknowns, and drafts. We can do our grooming together and for each other. We can see activities on the patio — visits from Robert Rabbit and Maudie's suitors. From a reclining position — we don't even have to raise our heads — we can see the birds at the feeder. Sometimes we see Cyril the squirrel plotting and planning how to get to the seeds by descending on the chain. We watched him fall to the ground once (he is not very careful). But, he doesn't give up! His Sylvia is not that adventurous.

In the early morning the sun shines on the chair. That is the very best time to complete major grooming processes, followed by a deep sleep. This is as good as in our basket over the heat register. If it is cold and stormy outside and Lip does not turn up the heat in the morning, we will use our basket but the best is our chair.

We can also see the TV from the chair. And, if someone comes to the door, we just have to sit up and lean forward and we can tell if it is someone important that requires our presence.

The chair is the centre of our universe.

While Lip was working we were willing to allow her to use the chair a few hours in the evening as we know she is tired and entitled to a few privileges around the house.

But, Auntie Jennifer, she is using the chair in the daytime! This is not acceptable and we are most upset. We have tried to tell her that she should not be watching daytime TV, anyway. This is a very bad habit and Lip does not need any more bad habits.

In the summer we are going to shop at garage sales and see if we can find a green plaid wing chair for Lip. This would solve all of our problems. In the meantime, we will ask for a board meeting with Lip so that we can come up with an acceptable chair schedule.

Last night Maudie fell off the TV again while she was sleeping.

She went SPLAT on the floor. Needless to say, we were very concerned. Lip and I checked her over very carefully and she is fine. Just a big loss of dignity.

We are praying for you, Auntie Jennifer. We hope that you are having comfortable naps and sleeps.

Love,
Maudie and Oliver

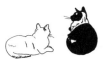

Letter #35 · It's A Fly Thing

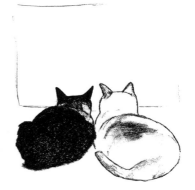

April 3, 2002

Dear Auntie Jennifer:

Spring should be here and it is not.

Now that Lip is home she has started on something called "spring cleaning." She and the cleaning ladies do cleaning all the time so we do not understand the spring part.

This is Oliver speaking.

Every year since we can remember the crocus beside the front step comes up the first day of spring. We are quite short sighted — Maudie more than I — and Lip takes great effort to show this to us from the dining room window. She said forget it this year. It came up one day and now has gone back to crocus winter land. But, we did hear the Canada geese the other day!

Lip said that they are back early because of the low value of the Canadian dollar.

Maudie has a new suitor. His name is Rodney. He is an older gentleman, with a black beard and long hair. He appears to be a little down on his luck. But, he is very dapper and works diligently on his grooming. He likes to sit in the parsley pot under the dining room window so he can gaze at Maudie and her provocative poses. I get quite concerned and anxious when Maudie does this. I know that her suitors have exotic thoughts on their minds, especially this time of the year.

When I get nervous about Maudie — her suitors, when she does a splat on the living room floor — I bite my nails. This causes Lip to chastise me about what a bad habit I am developing. That upsets me and then I get the hiccups. It is not easy living with Maudie and Lip, Auntie Jennifer.

The flies are back in the house. I guess that is a good sign that spring may be on its way. The other day, two of the flies were creating some intense energy on the sunlit floor in the living room. One fly was on the back of the other fly. Imagine! We found this very interesting. We asked Lip what they were doing.

She peered at them closely and said, "Um, they are... um... fornicating."

Fornicating? We have never heard of that. We asked Lip, "What is fornicating?"

Lip said, "I will tell you when you are older."

It must be a fly thing, Auntie Jennifer.

We know that you are very ill and we are praying for you everyday.

Love,
Oliver and Maudie

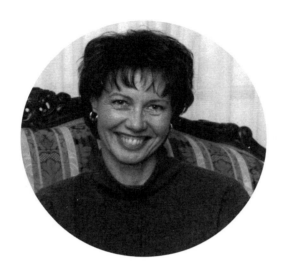

Jennifer Johnston
June 28, 1954 — April 3, 2002

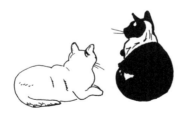